**DEVELOPED BY
BRAINBOTHY**

ABOUT THE AUTHOR

BrainBothy is a small business managed by a Psychological Therapist living in Scotland. She has chosen to remain anonymous as she currently still works full-time as a Cognitive Behavioural Psychological Therapist in the National Health Service, working in a service for older people living with dementia or other mental health conditions such as anxiety and depression.

She has over 10 years' experience working with older people and specialist training in dementia. BrainBothy is passionate about increasing access to safe and evidence-based information to support those living with and caring for people with dementia.

Outside of work, she loves to spend time in nature, walking or enjoying the fresh sea air. She also loves animals, particularly cats, and baking lovely cakes or as we say in Scotland 'funcy pieces' – something she inherited from her late Grandma.

ABOUT THIS RESOURCE BUNDLE.

This digital best seller is now available in print form!

This bundle includes:
Over 100 pages of dementia friendly resources.
About me document
Life story book
Communication cards
Days of the week posters
Food and drink flashcards
Memory aids
Routine cards for daily activities

Resources are dementia friendly, easy-to-read visual prompts to increase and maintain independence for adults living with dementia, memory loss or cognitive impairment.

This bundle does not replace formal treatment or therapy. If you are in need of additional support, please see your general practitioner or a professional.

HAVING A SHOWER

UNDRESS. REMOVE GLASSES & OTHER ACCESSORIES

TURN ON SHOWER & CHECK THE WATER TEMPERATURE

ENTER THE SHOWER. RINSE BODY & HAIR

1-2 PUMPS OF SHAMPOO. LATHER & RINSE HAIR

1-2 PUMPS SHOWER GEL OR SOAP. WASH FACE & BODY

RINSE WHOLE BODY

TURN OFF SHOWER & EXIT

DRY WITH A TOWEL

HAVING A SHOWER

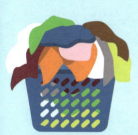

UNDRESS. REMOVE GLASSES & OTHER ACCESSORIES

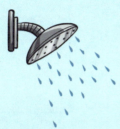

TURN ON SHOWER & CHECK THE TEMPERATURE

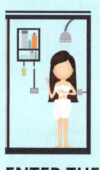

ENTER THE SHOWER. RINSE BODY & HAIR

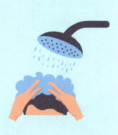

1-2 PUMPS OF SHAMPOO. LATHER & RINSE HAIR

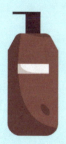

1-2 PUMPS SHOWER GEL OR SOAP. WASH FACE & BODY

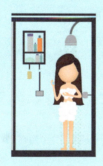

RINSE WHOLE BODY

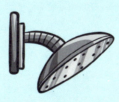

TURN OFF SHOWER & EXIT

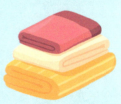

DRY WITH A TOWEL

USING THE TOILET

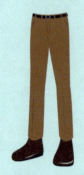 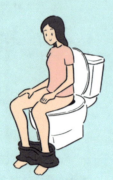 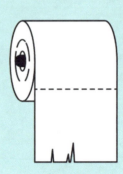 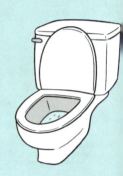

PULL DOWN UNDERWEAR AND BOTTOMS | **USE THE TOILET** | **WIPE & CLEAN USING TOILET ROLL** | **PUT USED TOILET ROLL IN THE TOILET**

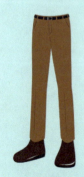 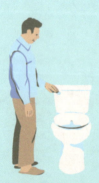 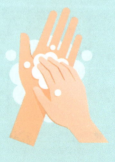 

PULL UP UNDERWEAR AND BOTTOMS | **FLUSH THE TOILET** | **WASH HANDS USING SOAP** | **DRY HANDS USING A TOWEL**

USING THE TOILET

PULL DOWN UNDERWEAR AND BOTTOMS

USE THE TOILET

WIPE & CLEAN USING TOILET ROLL

PUT USED TOILET ROLL IN THE TOILET

PULL UP UNDERWEAR AND BOTTOMS

FLUSH THE TOILET

WASH HANDS USING SOAP

DRY HANDS USING A TOWEL

BRUSHING TEETH

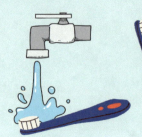 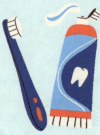 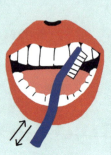 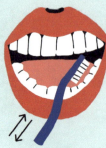

WET TOOTH BRUSH — **APPLY TOOTH PASTE** — **BRUSH TOP TEETH** — **BRUSH BOTTOM TEETH**

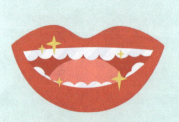 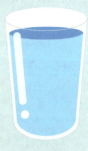 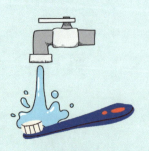

SPIT OUT TOOTH PASTE — **RINSE MOUTH WITH WATER** — **WASH TOOTH BRUSH**

BRUSHING TEETH

WET TOOTHBRUSH

APPLY TOOTHPASTE

BRUSH TOP TEETH, FRONT & BACK

BRUSH BOTTOM TEETH, FRONT & BACK

SPIT OUT TOOTHPASTE

RINSE MOUTH WITH WATER

WASH TOOTHBRUSH

RINSE WITH MOUTHWASH

MAKING TEA

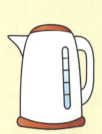 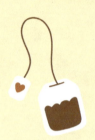 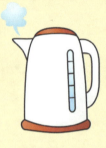 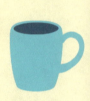

CHECK THE KETTLE AND FILL WITH WATER IF REQUIRED.　**PICK YOUR FAVOURITE MUG AND PUT A TEA BAG IN IT.**　**TURN ON KETTLE AND WAIT FOR IT TO BOIL.**　**ONCE BOILED CAREFULLY FILL YOUR MUG WITH HOT WATER**

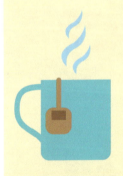 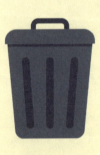 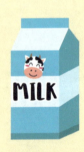 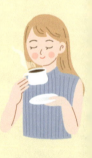

LEAVE THE TEABAG IN YOUR MUG FOR 3-5 MINUTES.　**REMOVE AND DISPOSE OF THE TEABAG.**　**ADD SUGAR OR MILK IF REQUIRED.**　**ENJOY!**

MAKING TEA

CHECK THE KETTLE AND FILL WITH WATER IF REQUIRED.

PICK YOUR FAVOURITE MUG AND PUT A TEA BAG IN IT.

TURN ON KETTLE AND WAIT FOR IT TO BOIL.

ONCE BOILED CAREFULLY FILL YOUR MUG WITH HOT WATER.

LEAVE THE TEABAG IN YOUR MUG FOR 3-5 MINUTES.

REMOVE AND DISPOSE OF THE TEABAG.

ADD SUGAR OR MILK IF REQUIRED.

ENJOY!

MAKING COFEE

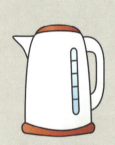 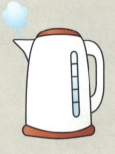 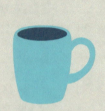 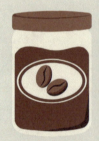

CHECK THE KETTLE AND FILL WITH WATER IF REQUIRED.

TURN ON KETTLE AND WAIT FOR IT TO BOIL.

PICK YOUR FAVOURITE MUG.

ADD COFFEE AND SUGAR IF REQUIRED

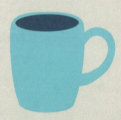 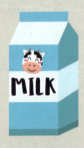 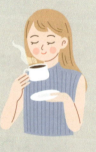

ONCE BOILED. CAREFULLY FILL YOUR MUG WITH HOT WATER.

ADD MILK IF REQUIRED AND STIR .

ENJOY!

MAKING COFFEE

CHECK THE KETTLE AND FILL WITH WATER IF REQUIRED.

TURN ON KETTLE AND WAIT FOR IT TO BOIL.

PICK YOUR FAVOURITE MUG.

ADD COFFEE AND SUGAR IF REQUIRED.

ONCE BOILED CAREFULLY FILL YOUR MUG WITH HOT WATER.

ADD MILK IF REQUIRED AND STIR.

ENJOY!

GETTING DRESSED

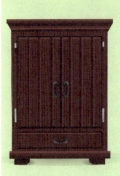
SELECT YOUR OUTFIT

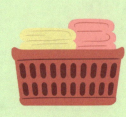
REMOVE CLOTHES YOU ARE WEARING

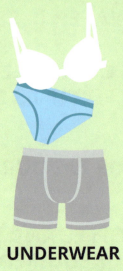
UNDERWEAR

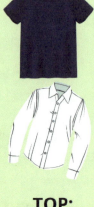
TOP: T-SHIRT, SHIRT

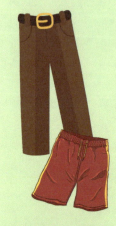
BOTTOMS: SKIRT, TROUSERS, SHORTS

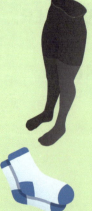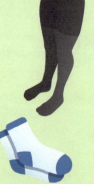
SOCKS OR TIGHTS

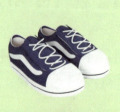
SLIPPERS OR SHOES

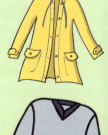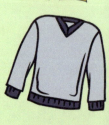
JUMPER, CARDIGAN OR COAT

GETTING DRESSED

SELECT YOUR OUTFIT

REMOVE CLOTHES YOU ARE WEARING

PUT ON UNDERWEAR

PUT ON A TOP: T-SHIRT OR SHIRT

PUT ON BOTTOMS: TROUSERS, SHORTS OR SKIRT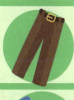

PUT ON SOCKS OR TIGHTS

PUT ON SHOES OR SLIPPERS

PUT ON A JUMPER, CARDIGAN OR JACKET

TIME FOR BED:

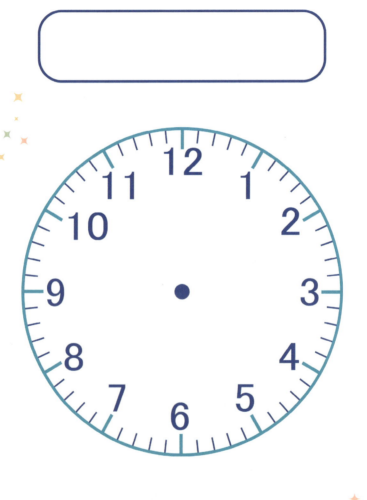

GET READY FOR BED:

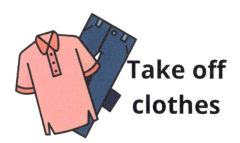 Take off clothes

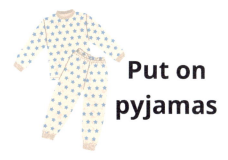 Put on pyjamas

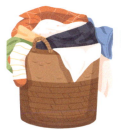 Put away dirty clothes

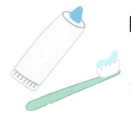 Brush your teeth

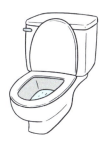 Go to the toilet

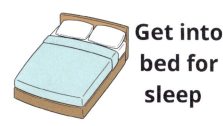 Get into bed for sleep

TODAY IS:

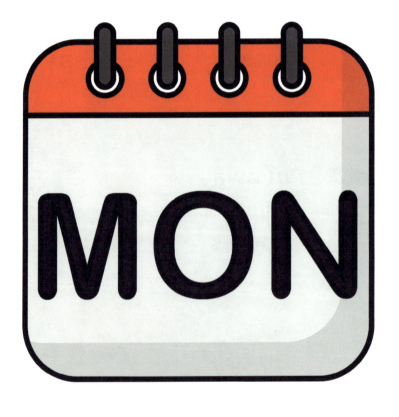

TODAY IS:

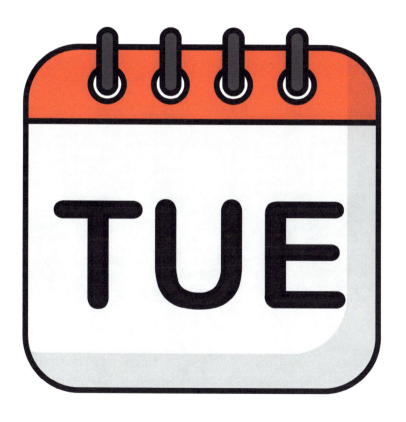

TODAY IS:

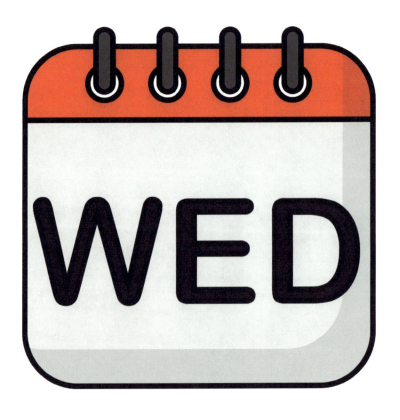

TODAY IS:

TODAY IS:

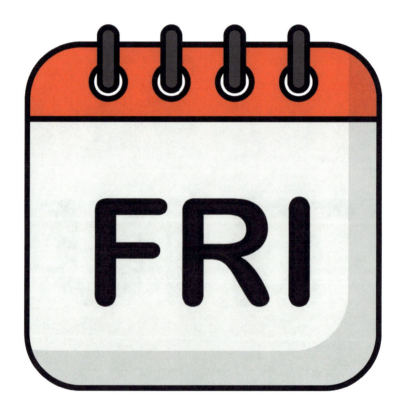

TODAY IS:

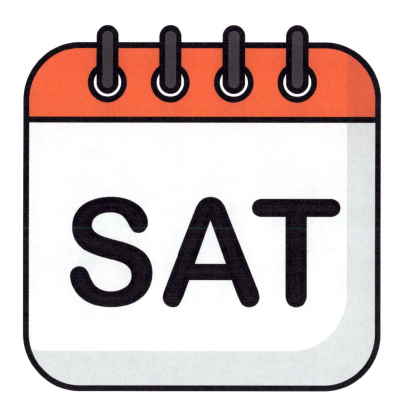

TODAY IS:

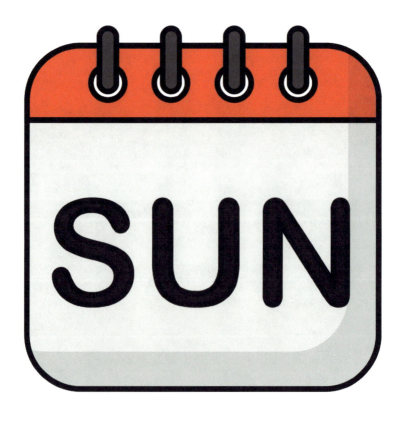

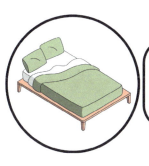 MY BEDROOM

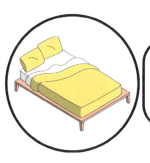 BEDROOM

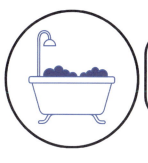 BATHROOM

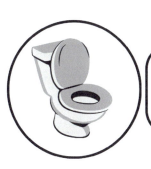 TOILET

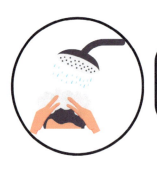 SHOWER ROOM

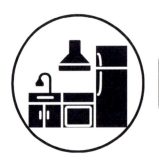 KITCHEN

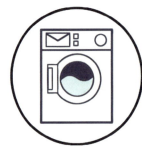 UTILITY ROOM

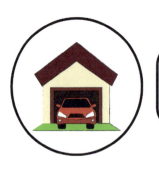 GARAGE

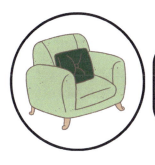 LIVING ROOM

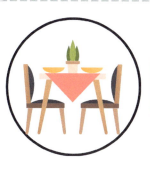 DINING ROOM

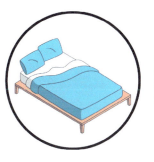 SPARE ROOM

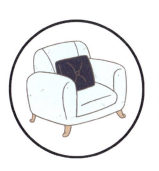 LOUNGE

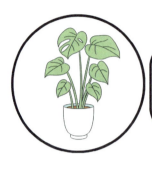 CONSERVATORY

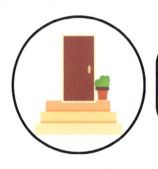 VESTIBULE

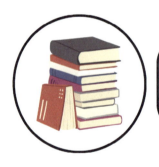 STUDY

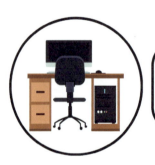 OFFICE

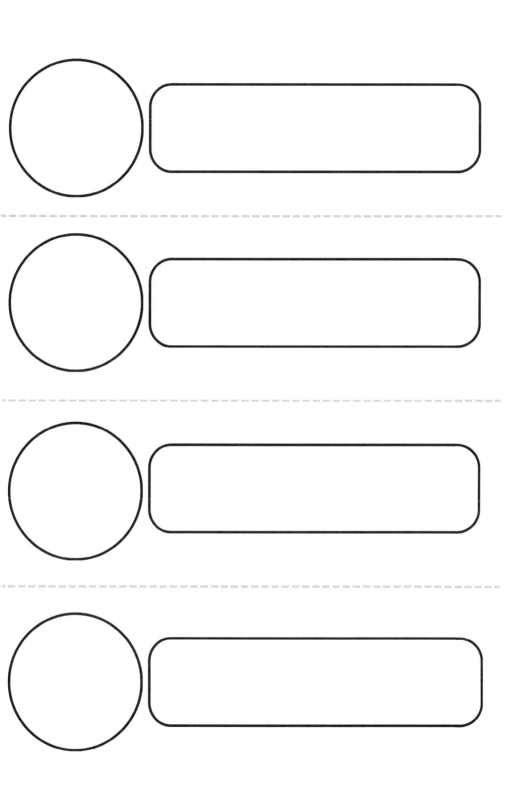

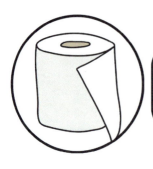 TOILET ROLL

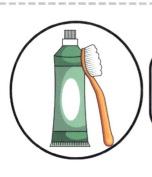 TOOTHBRUSH & TOOTHPASTE

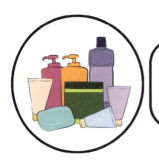 TOILETRIES

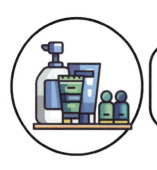 TOILETRIES

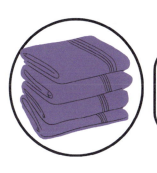 TOWELS

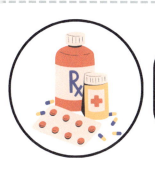 MEDICINE

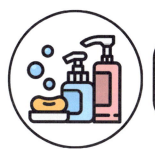 SHOWER GEL

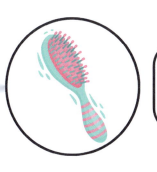 HAIR PRODUCTS

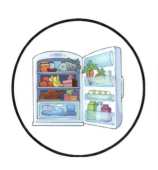 FRIDGE

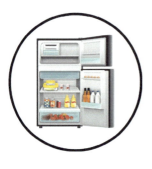 FREEZER

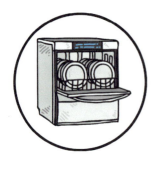 DISHWASHER

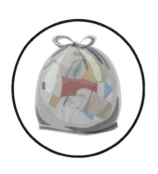 RUBBISH BIN

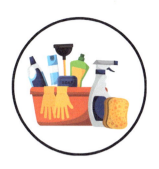 **CLEANING PRODUCTS**

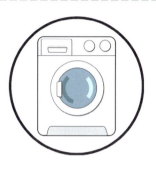 **WASHING MACHINE**

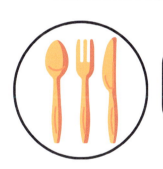 **CUTLERY**

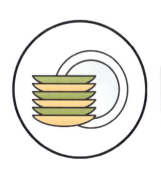 **PLATES**

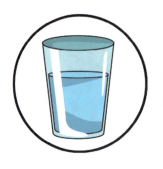 CUPS

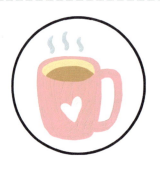 MUGS

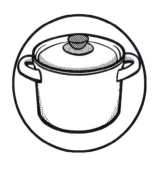 POTS & PANS

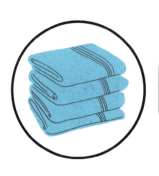 TEA TOWELS

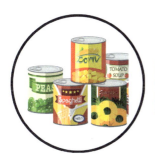 FOOD

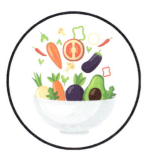 FOOD

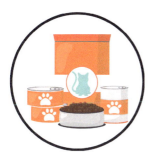 PET FOOD

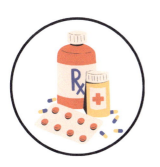 MEDICINE

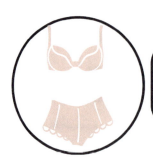 UNDERWEAR

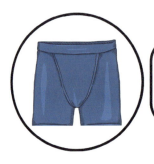 UNDERWEAR

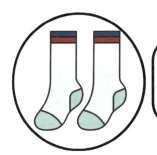 SOCKS

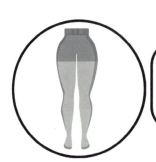 TIGHTS

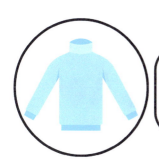 THERMAL

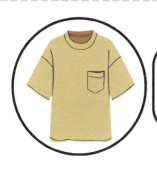 T-SHIRTS

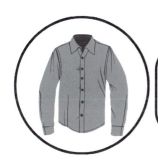 SHIRTS

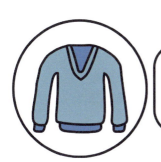 JUMPERS

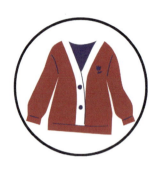 CARDIGAN

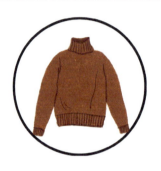 SWEATERS

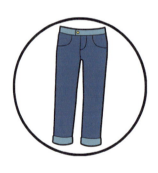 TROUSERS

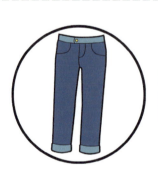 PANTS

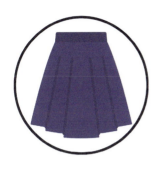 SKIRTS

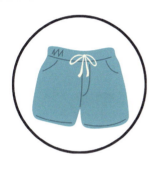 SHORTS

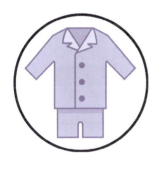 PYJAMMAS

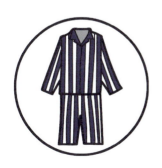 NIGHTWEAR

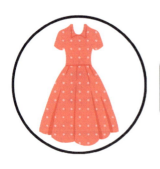 DRESSES

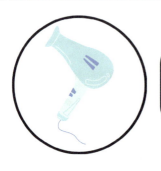 HAIR PRODUCTS

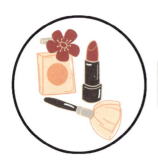 MAKE-UP

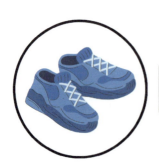 SHOES

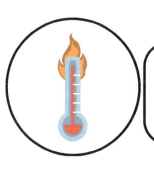 CAUTION: HOT WATER

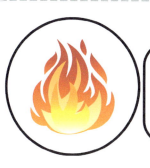 CAUTION: HOT SURFACE

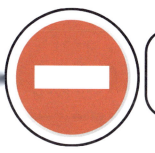 STOP: NO ENTRY

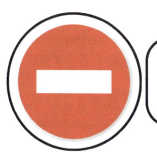 STOP: DO NOT TOUCH

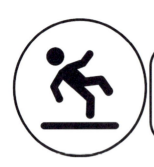 CAUTION: SLIPPERY

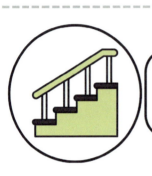 MIND THE STEP

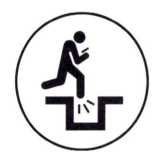 MIND THE GAP

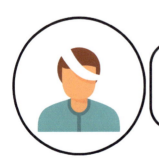 CAUTION: MIND YOUR HEAD

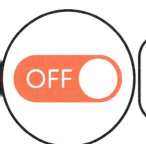 TURN OFF

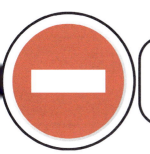 STOP: DO NOT OPEN

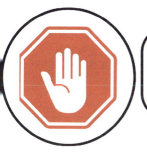 DO NOT USE

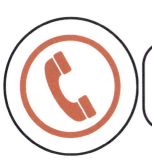 IN EMERGENCY CALL:

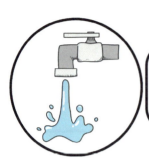 TURN OFF TAP

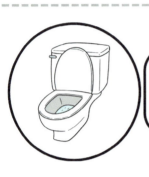 FLUSH THE TOILET

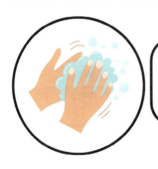 WASH HANDS WITH SOAP

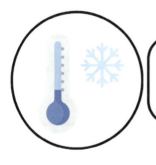 CAUTION: FREEZING

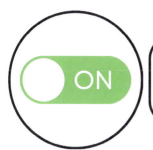 TURN ON

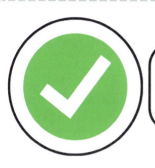 PLEASE USE

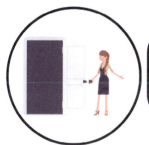 OPEN

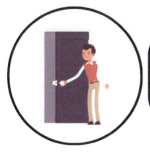 CLOSE

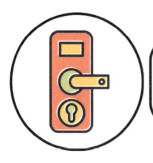 LOCK DOOR

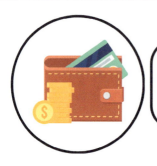 TAKE WALLET

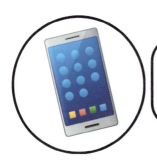 TAKE PHONE

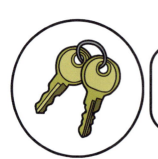 TAKE KEYS

About Me

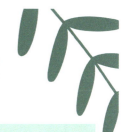

Photo here

My name:

Date of birth:

Important people:

I don't like...

My favourite...

Food:

Drink:

TV show:

Movie:

Music:

Hobby:

MY
LIFESTORY BOOK

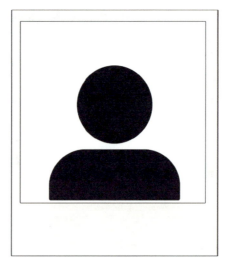

NAME:

I LIKE TO BE CALLED:

INTRODUCTION TO MY LIFE...

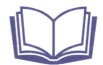

DATE OF BIRTH:

PLACE OF BIRTH:

FAMILY:

MOTHERS NAME & OCCUPATION:

FATHERS NAME & OCCUPATION:

POSITION IN FAMILY (E.G., OLDEST, YOUNGEST):

SIBLINGS NAMES (ELDEST FIRST):

OTHER FAMILY MEMBERS:

IMPORTANT PEOPLE

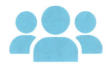

USE THIS PAGE TO DESCRIBE AND INCLUDE PHOTOS OF THE MOST IMPORTANT PEOPLE AND RELATIONSHIPS IN YOUR LIFE AND WHY THEY MATTER TO YOU. SUCH AS, PARTNER, CHILDREN, PARENTS, FRIENDS ETC.

OTHER RELATIONSHIPS

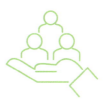

INCLUDE INFORMATION ABOUT OTHER RELATIONSHIPS THAT MATTER TO YOU IN THIS SECTION. SUCH AS: WIDER FAMILY, COLLEAGUES, NEIGHBOURS, PETS, CARERS, PEOPLE YOU ADMIRE.

MY
EARLY LIFE

**INCLUDE SIGNIFICANT MEMORIES FROM CHILDHOOD SUCH AS,
HOME LIFE, HOLIDAYS, GAMES, TOYS, MUSIC, HOBBIES, FRIENDS
AND MEMORIES FROM SCHOOL.
(INCLUDE PHOTOS).**

MY WORKING LIFE

INCLUDE INFORMATION ABOUT PRESENT AND PAST WORKING LIFE. FOR EXAMPLE, PLACES OF WORK, JOB TITLES, TRAINING AND QUALIFICATIONS, FIRST JOB, OTHER JOBS, WORKING RELATIONSHIPS. (INCLUDE PHOTOS, CERTIFICATES ETC.)

PLACES THAT MATTER TO ME

INCLUDE INFORMATION ABOUT PRESENT AND PAST WORKING LIFE. FOR EXAMPLE, PLACES OF WORK, JOB TITLES, TRAINING AND QUALIFICATIONS, FIRST JOB, OTHER JOBS, WORKING RELATIONSHIPS. (INCLUDE PHOTOS, CERTIFICATES ETC.)

SIGNIFICANT LIFE EVENTS

DESCRIBE SIGNIFICANT OCCASIONS OR EVENTS THAT HAVE HAD AN IMPACT ON YOUR LIFE. THIS MIGHT INCLDUE, PASSING DRIVING TEST, GRADUATION, MEETING PARTNER, WEDDING DAY, BIRTH OF CHILD / GRANDCHILD, MOVING HOME, BEREAVEMENT ETC.

MY LATER LIFE

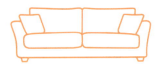

THINGS YOU WOULD LIKE PEOPLE TO KNOW ABOUT YOUR LATER LIFE. CONSIDER HOW THINGS HAVE CHANGES AS YOU GROW OLDER SUCH AS, WHEN AND WHY YOU RETIRED, HOW YOU SPEND YOUR TIME, WHAT DO YOU ENJOY OR DISLIKE ABOUT GROWING OLDER.

MY LIFESTYLE NOW

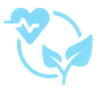

WHAT DO YOU LIKE TO TALK ABOUT? ARE THERE TOPICS YOU LIKE TO AVOID? HOW DO YOU RELAX? HOW DO YOU LIKE TO SPEND YOUR TIME AND WITH WHO? WHAT ARE YOUR DAILY ROUTINES LIKE? WHAT ROUTINES ARE IMPORTANT?

MY LIFESTYLE: SEXUALITY

HOW WOULD YOU DESCRIBE YOUR SEXUAL AND GENDER IDENTITY? WHAT PRONOUNS DO YOU USE?

MY LIFESTYLE: BELIEFS

WHAT IS YOU RELIGION / FAITH (IF ANY)? DO YOU ATTEND A PLACE OF WORSHIP? DO YOU FOLLOW ANY SPIRITUAL PRACTICES? DO YOU NEED SUPPORT TO FOLLOW YOUR BELIEFS? WHAT ARE YOUR POLICITCAL BELIEFS?

LIKES & DISLIKES: ACTIVITY

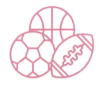

RECORD INFORMATION ABOUT ACTIVITIES, INTERESTS, HOBBIES THAT YOU ENJOY OR DISLIKE. THIS MIGHT INCLDUE CURRENT HOBBIES, SPORTS TEAMS YOU SUPPORT, OUTINGS OR GROUPS YOU ENJOY OR THINGS YOU WOULD LIKE TO TRY.

LIKES & DISLIKES: MUSIC

RECORD YOUR MUSIC PREFERENCES HERE. WHAT GENRE DO YOU LIKE / DISLIKE? DO YOU HAVE A FAVOURITE ARTIST? DO YOU PLAY AN INSTRUMENT? HOW AND WHEN DO YOU LIKE TO LISTEN TO MUSIC? DO YOU ENJOY THE RADIO OR LIVE MUSIC?

LIKES & DISLIKES: TV & FILM

RECORD INFORMATION ABOUT TV AND FILMS THAT YOU DO / DON'T ENJOY. FOR EXAMPLE, WHAT ARE YOU FAVOURITE TV SHOWS AND FILMS? WHAT GENRES DO YOU LIKE BEST? ARE THERE ANY YOU DON'T LIKE? DO YOU NEED SUPPORT TO WATCH TV?

LIKES & DISLIKES: PERSONAL CARE

RECORD YOUR APPEARANCE AND PERSONAL CARE PREFERENCES HERE. WHAT DO YOU LIKE TO WEAR? DO YOU WEAR ANY RELIGIOUS ITEMS? WHAT DO YOU LIKE TO WEAR AT NIGHT? WHAT COSMETICS & TOILETIRES DO YOU LIKE? HOW DO YOU LIKE TO HAVE YOUR (FACIAL) HAIR? DO LIKE TO HAVE MAKE-UP / NAILS DONE?

LIKES & DISLIKES: FOOD & DRINK

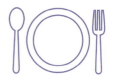

RECORD INFORMATION ABOUT FOOD & DRINK PREFERENCES. WHAT DO YOU LIKE / DISLIKE? DO YOU NEED SUPPORT TO EAT / DRINK? DO YOU HAVE ANY ALLERGIES OR INTOLERANCES? DO YOU LIKE TO GO OUT FOR FOOD & DRINK? DO YOU LIKE TO COOK?

MY WISHES FOR THE FUTURE

RECORD YOUR WISHES ABOUT YOUR FUTURE CARE. WHERE WOULD YOU LIKE TO BE CARE FOR (OWN HOME / CARE HOME ETC.)? WHO WOULD YOU LIKE TO CARE FOR YOU? WHO WOULD YOU WANT TO MAKE DECISIONS FOR YOU? DO YOU HAVE A WILL? WISHES AT YOUR END OF LIFE SUCH AS FUNERAL ARRANGEMENTS.

ADDITIONAL INFORMATION

I WANT...

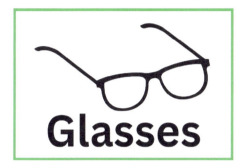 Glasses	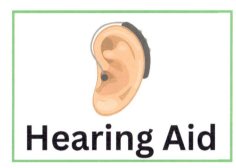 Hearing Aid
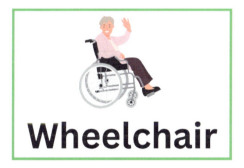 Wheelchair	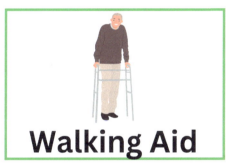 Walking Aid
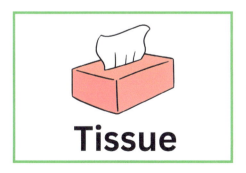 Tissue	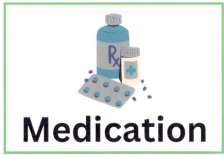 Medication

I WANT...

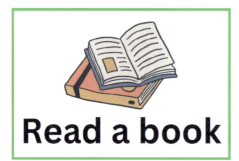
Read a book

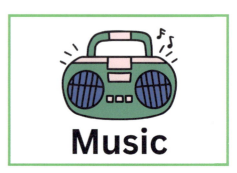
Music

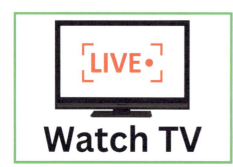
Watch TV

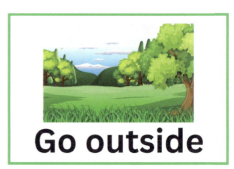
Go outside

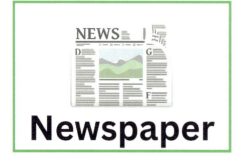
Newspaper

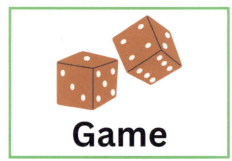
Game

I WANT...

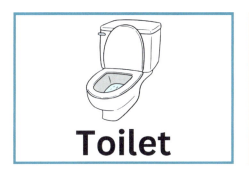
Toilet

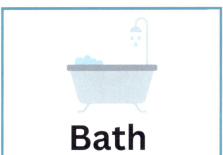
Bath

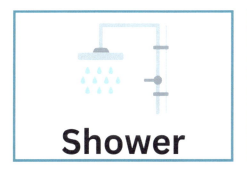
Shower

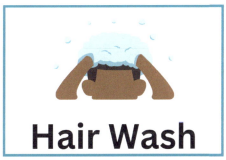
Hair Wash

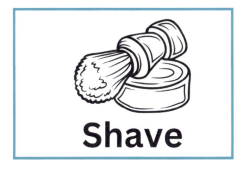
Shave

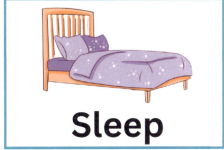
Sleep

I WANT...

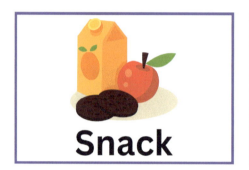
Snack

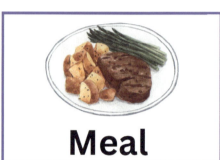
Meal

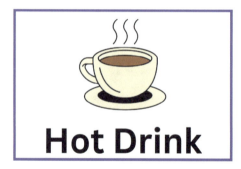
Hot Drink

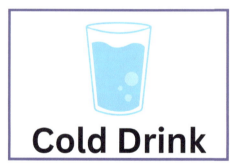
Cold Drink

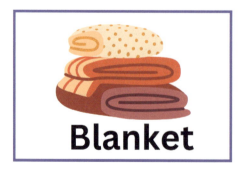
Blanket

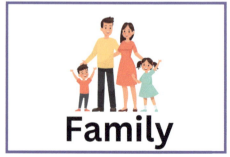
Family

I FEEL...

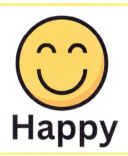 **Happy**	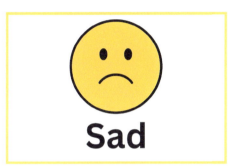 **Sad**
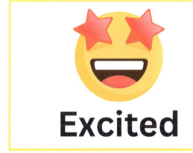 **Excited**	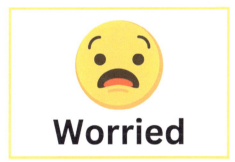 **Worried**
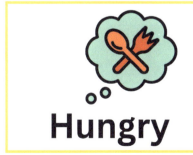 **Hungry**	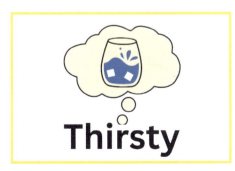 **Thirsty**

I FEEL...

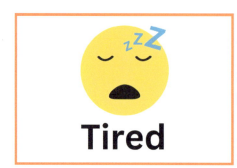
Tired

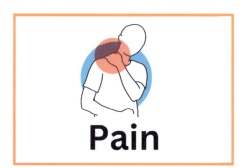
Pain

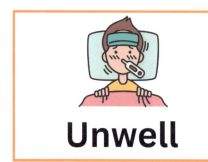
Unwell

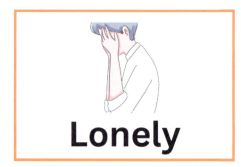
Lonely

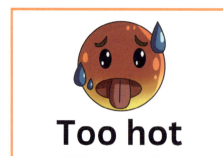
Too hot

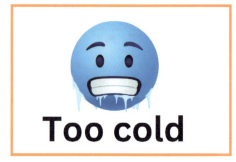
Too cold

I FEEL...

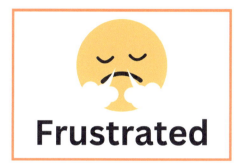
Frustrated

Scared

Anxious

Surprised

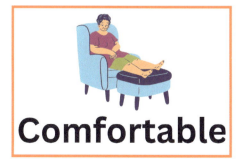
Comfortable

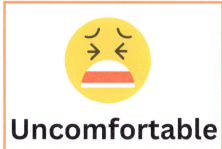
Uncomfortable

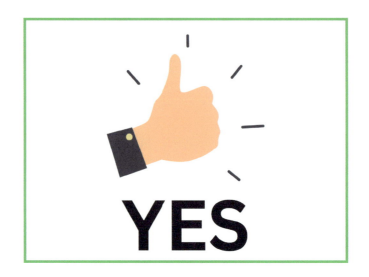

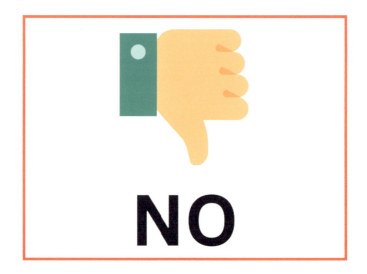

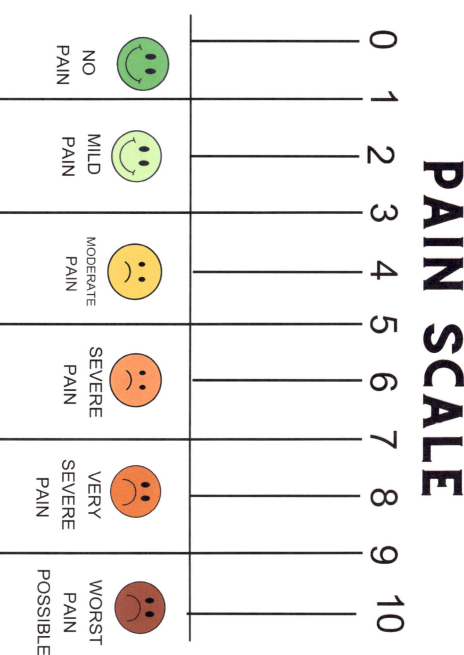

WHERE IT HURTS

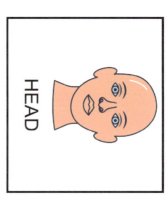

HEAD

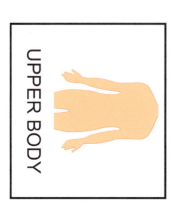

UPPER BODY

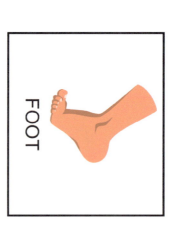

FOOT

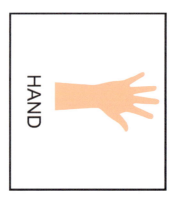

LOWER BODY

HAND

WHERE IT HURTS

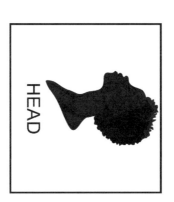

HEAD

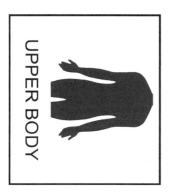

UPPER BODY

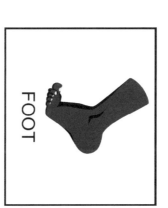

FOOT

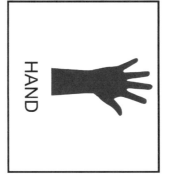

HAND

LOWER BODY

WHERE IT HURTS
HEAD / FACE PAIN

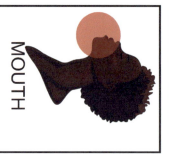

MOUTH

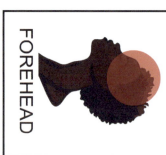

FOREHEAD

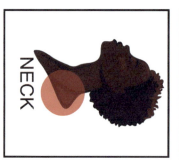

THROAT

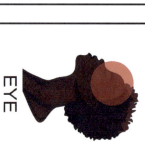

EYE

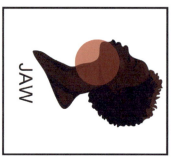

NECK

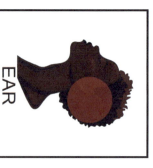

EAR

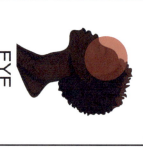

JAW

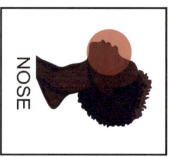

NOSE

WHERE IT HURTS
HEAD / FACE PAIN

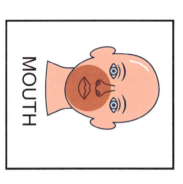
MOUTH

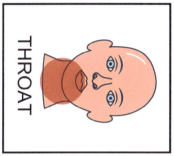
THROAT

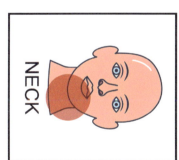
NECK

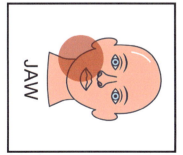
JAW

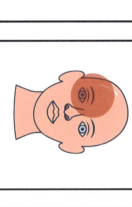
FOREHEAD

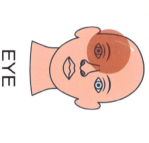
EYE

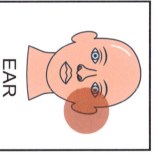
EAR

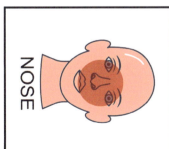
NOSE

WHERE IT HURTS
UPPER BODY

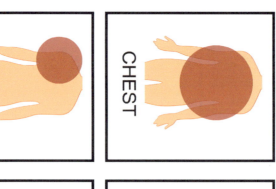
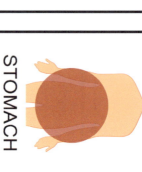
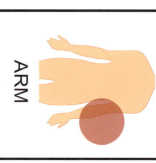
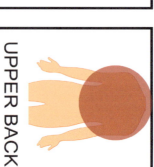
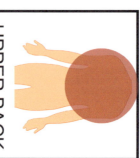
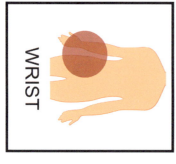
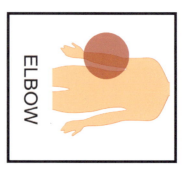
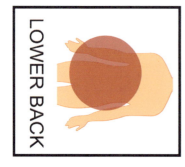

- SHOULDER
- CHEST
- ARM
- STOMACH
- WRIST
- UPPER BACK
- LOWER BACK
- ELBOW

WHERE IT HURTS
UPPER BODY

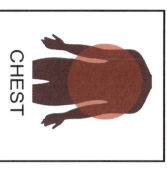 SHOULDER	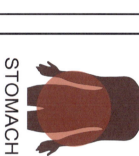 CHEST
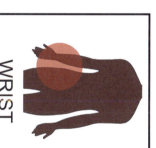 ARM	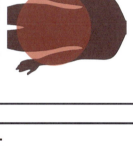 STOMACH
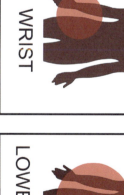 WRIST	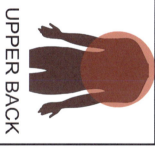 UPPER BACK
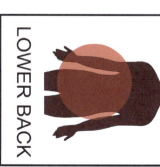 LOWER BACK	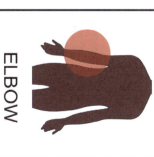 ELBOW

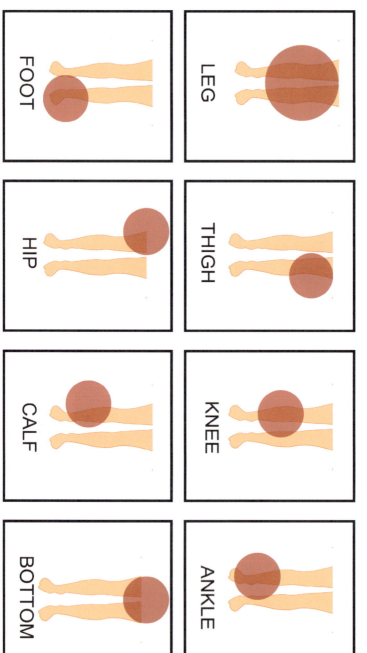

WHERE IT HURTS
LOWER BODY

- FOOT
- LEG
- HIP
- THIGH
- CALF
- KNEE
- BOTTOM
- ANKLE

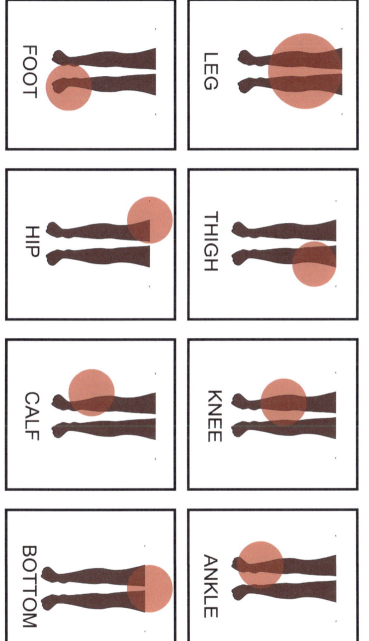

WHERE IT HURTS
HAND PAIN

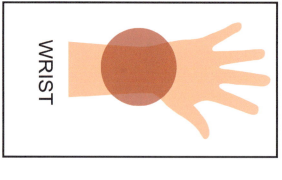
WRIST

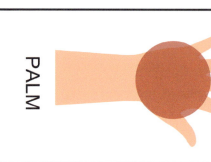
PALM

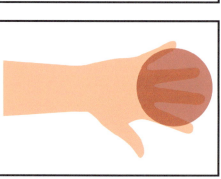
FINGERS

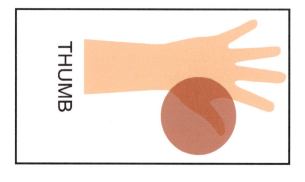
THUMB

WHERE IT HURTS
HAND PAIN

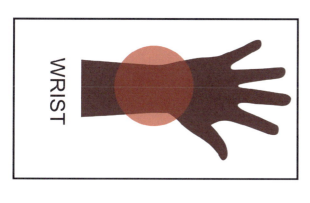

WRIST

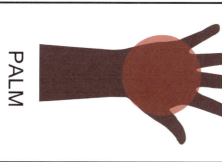

PALM

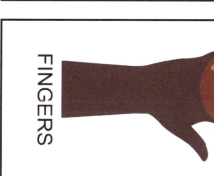

FINGERS

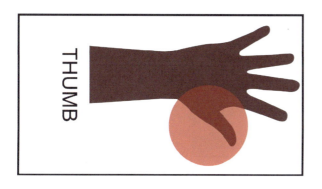

THUMB

WHERE IT HURTS
FOOT PAIN

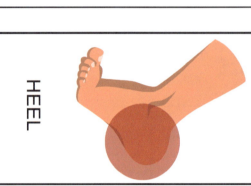

FOOT

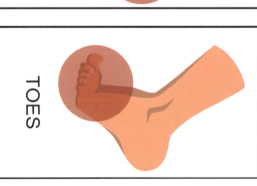

HEEL

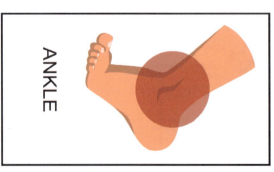

TOES

ANKLE

WHERE IT HURTS

FOOT PAIN

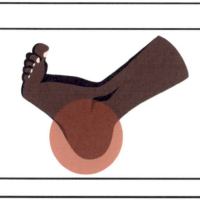

FOOT

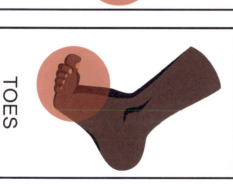

HEEL

TOES

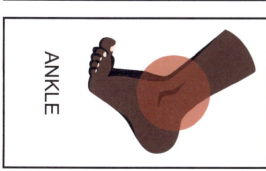

ANKLE

WHERE IT HURTS

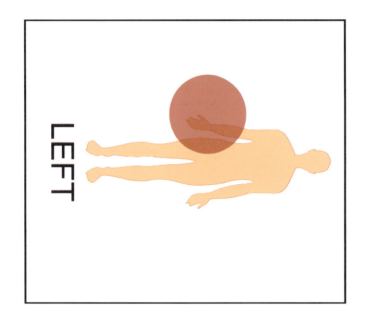

LEFT

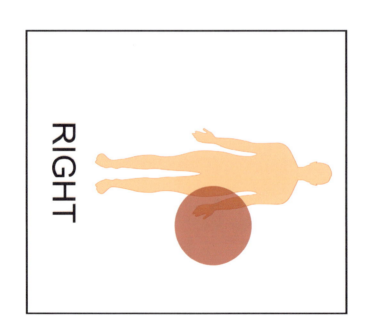

RIGHT

WHERE IT HURTS

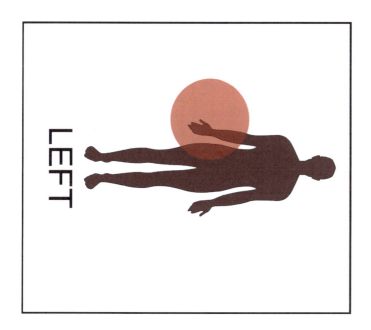

LEFT

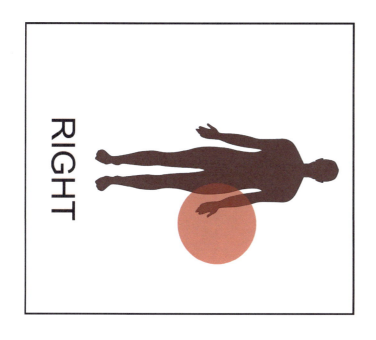

RIGHT

Personal care checklist

	Monday	Tuesday	Wednesday	Thursday	Friday	Saturday	Sunday
Brush and floss teeth.							
Shower or bathe using soap or gel.							
Wash hair with shampoo.							
Dry body, & hair with a towel or hairdryer.							
Put on clean clothes, underwear and socks.							
Take medication as prescribed.							
Prepare and eat breakfast, lunch and dinner.							

Personal care checklist

		M	T	W	T	F	S	S
	Brush and floss teeth.							
	Shower or bathe using soap or gel.							
	Wash hair with shampoo.							
	Dry body & hair with a towel or hairdryer.							
	Put on clean clothes, underwear and socks.							
	Take medication as prescribed.							
	Prepare and eat breakfast, lunch and dinner.							

Personal care checklist

	Monday	Tuesday	Wednesday	Thursday	Friday	Saturday	Sunday

WEEKLY PLANNER

	AM	PM
MONDAY		
TUESDAY		
WEDNESDAY		
THURSDAY		
FRIDAY		
SATURDAY		
SUNDAY		

TODAY

DAY:

DATE:

MONTH:

WEATHER:

I AM:

I WANT...

Hot Food
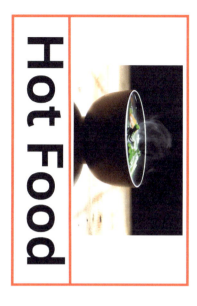

Hot Drink
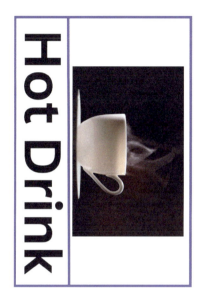

Snack
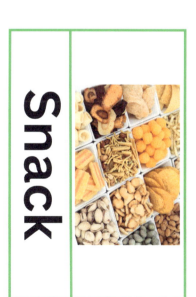

Cold Drink
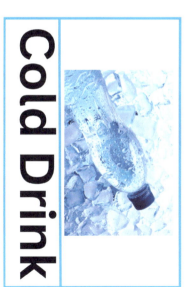

SNACKS

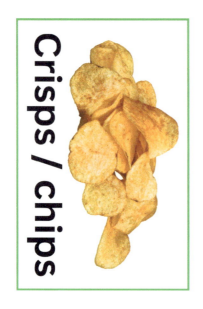

Crisps / chips

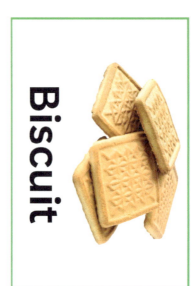

Biscuit

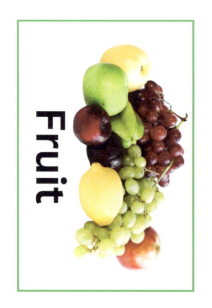

Fruit

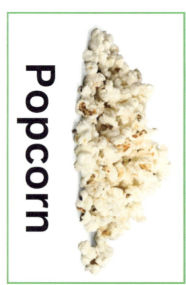

Popcorn

SNACKS

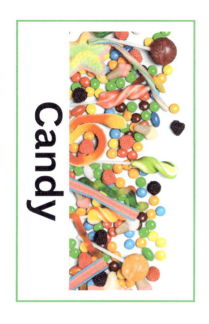

Candy

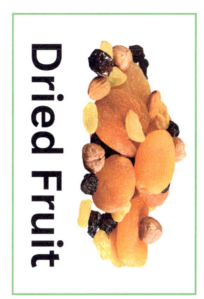

Dried Fruit

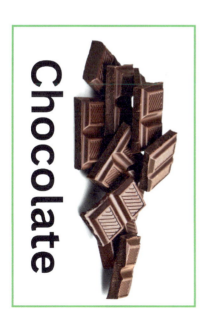

Chocolate

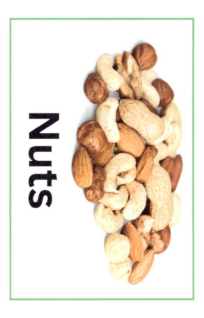

Nuts

SNACKS

Crackers

Jelly / Jello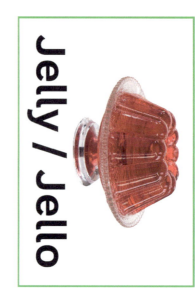

Yoghurt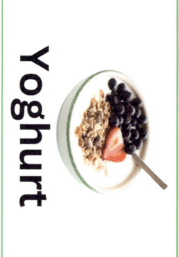

COLD DRINKS

Fruit Juice
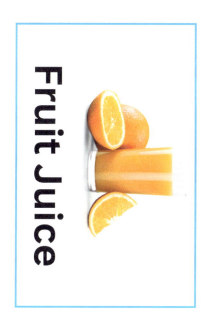

Water
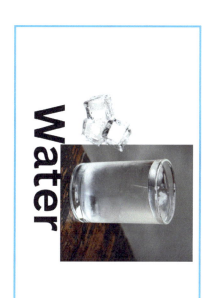

Squash
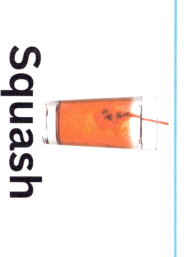

Iced Tea
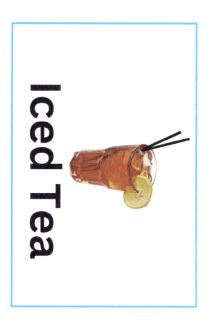

COLD DRINKS

Soda

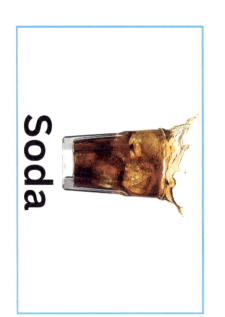

Iced Coffee

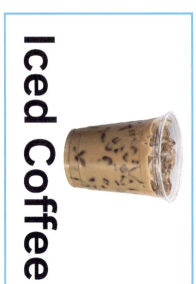

Milkshake

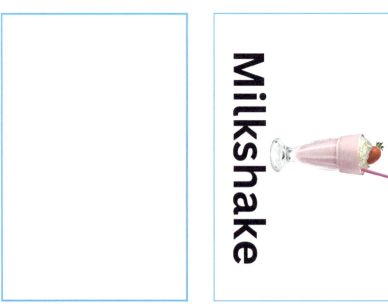

HOT DRINKS

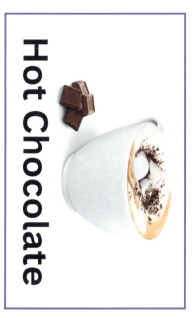
Hot Chocolate

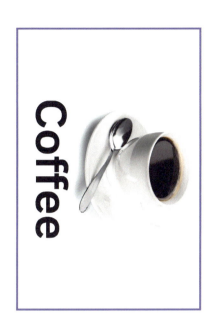
Coffee

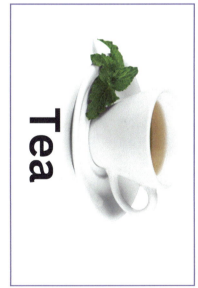
Tea

HOT FOODS

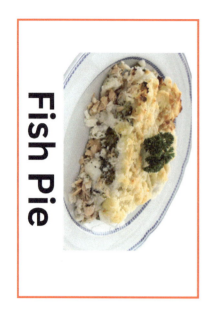
Fish Pie

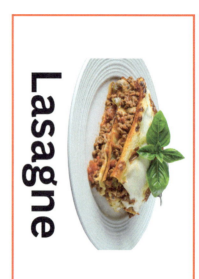
Lasagne

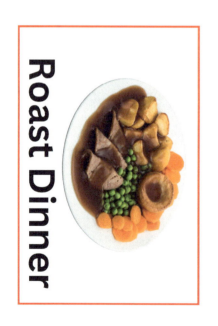
Roast Dinner

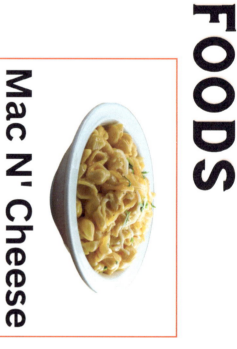
Mac N' Cheese

HOT FOODS

Curry
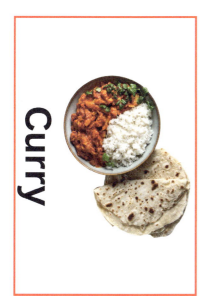

Burger
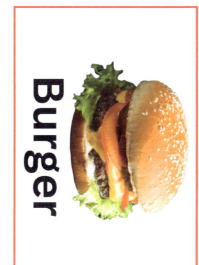

Omlette
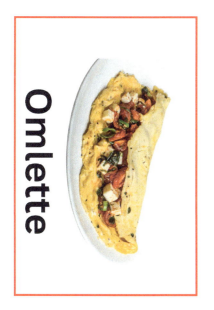

Soup
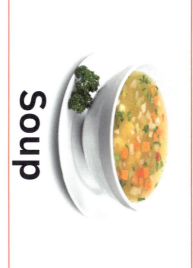

HOT FOODS

Bolognese
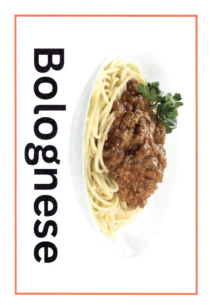

Stir-fry
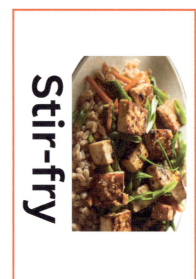

Fish & chips
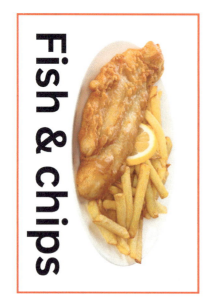

Stew
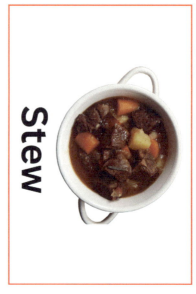

HOT FOODS

Steak

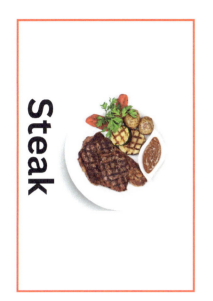

Chilli

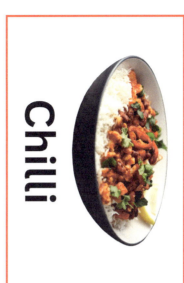

Pizza

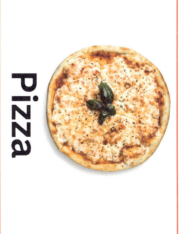

Meal Planner

Monday
- [ ] BREAKFAST :
- [ ] LUNCH :
- [ ] DINNER :

Tuesday
- [ ] BREAKFAST :
- [ ] LUNCH :
- [ ] DINNER :

Wednesday
- [ ] BREAKFAST :
- [ ] LUNCH :
- [ ] DINNER :

Thursday
- [ ] BREAKFAST :
- [ ] LUNCH :
- [ ] DINNER :

Friday
- [ ] BREAKFAST :
- [ ] LUNCH :
- [ ] DINNER :

Saturday
- [ ] BREAKFAST :
- [ ] LUNCH :
- [ ] DINNER :

Sunday
- [ ] BREAKFAST :
- [ ] LUNCH :
- [ ] DINNER :

Shopping List

- [x] Tick the box after you have eaten the meal each day
- [ ]
- [ ]

HAVE I EATEN MY MEALS?

MONDAY
- [ ] Breakfast
- [ ] Lunch
- [ ] Dinner

TUESDAY
- [ ] Breakfast
- [ ] Lunch
- [ ] Dinner

WEDNESDAY
- [ ] Breakfast
- [ ] Lunch
- [ ] Dinner

THURSDAY
- [ ] Breakfast
- [ ] Lunch
- [ ] Dinner

FRIDAY
- [ ] Breakfast
- [ ] Lunch
- [ ] Dinner

SATURDAY
- [ ] Breakfast
- [ ] Lunch
- [ ] Dinner

SUNDAY
- [ ] Breakfast
- [ ] Lunch
- [ ] Dinner

AM I DRINKING ENOUGH WATER?

MONDAY
- ☐ 1 LITRE
- ☐ 2 LITRES
- ☐ 3 LITRES

TUESDAY
- ☐ 1 LITRE
- ☐ 2 LITRES
- ☐ 3 LITRES

WEDNESDAY
- ☐ 1 LITRE
- ☐ 2 LITRES
- ☐ 3 LITRES

THURSDAY
- ☐ 1 LITRE
- ☐ 2 LITRES
- ☐ 3 LITRES

FRIDAY
- ☐ 1 LITRE
- ☐ 2 LITRES
- ☐ 3 LITRES

SATURDAY
- ☐ 1 LITRE
- ☐ 2 LITRES
- ☐ 3 LITRES

SUNDAY
- ☐ 1 LITRE
- ☐ 2 LITRES
- ☐ 3 LITRES

MEDICATION LIST

DATE: _____

#	MEDICATION	I TAKE IT FOR	DOSE	DIRECTIONS
1				
2				
3				
4				
5				
6				
7				
8				
9				
10				
11				
12				
13				
14				
15				
16				
17				
18				
19				
20				

MEDICATION CHECKLIST

NAME:

WEEK COMMENCING:

MEDICATION & DOSE	TIME TAKEN	M	T	W	T	F	S	S

TICK THE BOX AFTER YOU HAVE TAKEN YOUR MEDICATION

MEDICATION CHECKLIST

WEEK COMMENCING:

AM Medication & dose	Time Taken	M	T	W	T	F	S	S

PM Medication & dose	Time Taken	M	T	W	T	F	S	S

Other Medication	Time Taken	M	T	W	T	F	S	S

HAVE I TAKEN MY MEDICATION?

MONDAY
- ☐ MORNING
- ☐ AFTERNOON

TUESDAY
- ☐ MORNING
- ☐ AFTERNOON

WEDNESDAY
- ☐ MORNING
- ☐ AFTERNOON

THURSDAY
- ☐ MORNING
- ☐ AFTERNOON

FRIDAY
- ☐ MORNING
- ☐ AFTERNOON

SATURDAY
- ☐ MORNING
- ☐ AFTERNOON

SUNDAY
- ☐ MORNING
- ☐ AFTERNOON

MY CARE CHECKLIST

NAME:

WEEK COMMENCING:

CHECKLIST ITEM	TIME	M	T	W	T	F	S	S
WAKE UP & GO TO TOILET								
BRUSH & FLOSS TEETH								
PREPARE & EAT BREAKFAST								
MORNING MEDICATION								
BATH OR SHOWER								
WASH HAIR								
DRY BODY & HAIR								
CHANGE INTO CLEAN CLOTHES & UNDERWEAR								
PREPARE & EAT LUNCH								
AFTERNOON MEDICATION								
CLEAN DISHES								
WASH CLOTHES								
FEED PET								
CHANGE BEDDING								
PREPARE & EAT DINNER								
EVENING MEDICATION								
CHANGE INTO CLEAN PYJAMAS								
BRUSH & FLOSS TEETH BEFORE BED								
ENSURE DOORS ARE LOCKED								
DRINK WATER								

HAVE I SHOWERED OR BATHED?

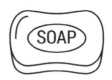

MONDAY
- [ ] Body
- [ ] Hair wash

TUESDAY
- [ ] Body
- [ ] Hair wash

WEDNESDAY
- [ ] Body
- [ ] Hair wash

THURSDAY
- [ ] Body
- [ ] Hair wash

FRIDAY
- [ ] Body
- [ ] Hair wash

SATURDAY
- [ ] Body
- [ ] Hair wash

SUNDAY
- [ ] Body
- [ ] Hair wash

HAVE I BRUSHED MY TEETH?

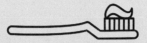

MONDAY
- ☐ MORNING
- ☐ EVENING

TUESDAY
- ☐ MORNING
- ☐ EVENING

WEDNESDAY
- ☐ MORNING
- ☐ EVENING

THURSDAY
- ☐ MORNING
- ☐ EVENING

FRIDAY
- ☐ MORNING
- ☐ EVENING

SATURDAY
- ☐ MORNING
- ☐ EVENING

SUNDAY
- ☐ MORNING
- ☐ EVENING

HAVE I BEEN PHYSICALLY ACTIVE?

MONDAY
- ☐ MORNING
- ☐ AFTERNOON

TUESDAY
- ☐ MORNING
- ☐ AFTERNOON

WEDNESDAY
- ☐ MORNING
- ☐ AFTERNOON

THURSDAY
- ☐ MORNING
- ☐ AFTERNOON

FRIDAY
- ☐ MORNING
- ☐ AFTERNOON

SATURDAY
- ☐ MORNING
- ☐ AFTERNOON

SUNDAY
- ☐ MORNING
- ☐ AFTERNOON

THIS RESOURCE GUIDE IS A PRODUCT DEVELOPED BY BRAINBOTHY

FOR MORE RESOURCES, FIND US ON:
ETSY
AMAZON
INSTAGRAM

CONSISTENTLY RATED

REPRODUCTION RIGHTS DO NOT TRANSFER WITH SALE.
ANY FORM OF DUPLICATION, DISTRIBUTION OR RESELLING FOR COMMERCIAL PURPOSES IS PROHIBITED.
THIS ITEM IS FOR YOUR PERSONAL USE ONLY.

Manufactured by Amazon.ca
Bolton, ON